Sundays with Matthew

A Young Boy with Autism and
an Artist Share Their Sketchbooks

Sundays with Matthew

A Young Boy with Autism and an Artist Share Their Sketchbooks

Foreword by
Elisa Gagnon

Written & Illustrated by
Matthew Lancelle & Jeanette Lesada

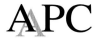

Autism Asperger Publishing Co.
P.O. Box 23173
Shawnee Mission, Kansas 66283-0173
www.asperger.net

© 2006 by Autism Asperger Publishing Co.
P.O. Box 23173
Shawnee Mission, Kansas 66283-0173
www.asperger.net

Lancelle, Matthew.
　　Sundays with Matthew : a young boy with autism and an artist share their sketchbooks /
　　written & illustrated by Matthew Lancelle & Jeanette Lesada. -- 1st ed. -- Shawnee Mission, KS :
　　Autism Asperger Pub. Co., 2006.

　　　　p. ; cm.

　　　　LCCN 2005934401
　　　　ISBN-13: 978-1-931282-84-0 (pbk.)
　　　　ISBN-10: 1-931282-84-6 (pbk.)
　　　　Audience: children grades 3-5 and their parents and teachers.

　　　　1. Autism in children--Juvenile literature. 2. Autistic children--Juvenile literature.
　　3. Art therapy for children--Juvenile literature. 4. Imagery (Psychology) in children--Juvenile literature.
　　5. Child development--Juvenile literature. 6. Developmentally disabled children--Means of communication--
　　Juvenile literature. 7. Children's drawings--Juvenile literature. I. Lesada, Jeanette. II. Title.

RJ506.A9 L36 2006　　　　　　　　　　　　　　2005934401
618.92/85882--dc22　　　　　　　　　　　　　　0512

This book is designed in American Typewriter and Typewriter Oldstyle.

Printed in South Korea.

FOREWORD

People with autism are commonly thought of as living in a world of their own, cut off from typical social interaction. At first glance this may seem to be true, but those who know people with autism sometimes find ways to achieve meaningful connections in nonconventional ways.

Years ago I was teaching children with autism in a laboratory classroom setting. Students were placed in this hospital-based school when they were not experiencing success in their community school and when their behaviors interfered significantly with their ability to learn. One of my students was a gifted artist, and even though he was a child with few words, the figures he created from play dough were truly remarkable, detailed and life-like. It was obvious that he had a gift, and I had no idea how to help him develop his talent.

Fortunately, a gifted local artist, Myrna Minnis, also known as the Oogly Lady, volunteered to work with this student. Every week for more than a year, she came to my classroom to work alongside the student. Over time, she taught him to use different kinds of clay and to incorporate new techniques into his art. In the process, I watched a relationship grow between the veteran and the emerging artist that is the type of relationship that can only develop between people who share a common passion. As they continued to work together, the student experienced much more than art lessons: His verbal language increased and his behaviors improved. He became much more focused and was eventually able to return to a public school setting. The art time with Myrna was a key factor in the student's improved behavior and his ability to become a valued and contributing member of the community.

Using a special interest and talent is a proven way to help a child reach his or her full potential. Since children and youth with autism often have well-defined special interests, it is valuable to determine what those interests are and find ways to use them to reinforce appropriate behavior. For instance, if a child is interested in dinosaurs, a trip to the dinosaur exhibit at the museum would be a motivating reward for a job well done. Even more important, however, is incorporating the special interest into the child's learning environment. For example, a child interested in dinosaurs may suddenly be interested in math when he is counting dinosaurs or doing a word problem that incorporates dinosaurs into the equation.

Sundays with Matthew is a wonderful example of a special relationship between two artists sharing a passion for art and also for life. Jeanette incorporates Matthew's love of monsters and sea creatures into their art time and also uses the time to teach emotions and appropriate social interactions. The drawings are used to spark conversation and to help Jeanette and Matthew communicate. The sketchbook tips in the back of the book can be used to help others use this technique when working with children and youth with autism.

The relationship between Jeanette and Matthew portrayed in this unique book is sure to warm your heart. Their shared interest in drawing has led to a friendship that will inspire others to look for commonalities instead of differences in people.

> – Elisa Gagnon, author, *Power Cards: Using Special Interests to Motivate Children and Youth with Asperger Syndrome and Autism,* co-author, *This Is Asperger Syndrome*

Hello There!

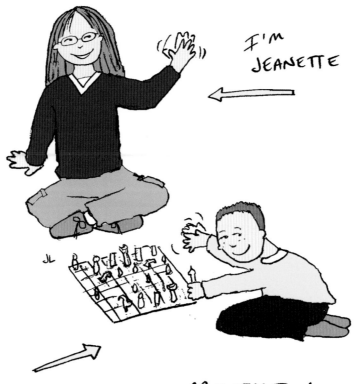

Welcome to Sundays
with Matthew!

Matthew is ...

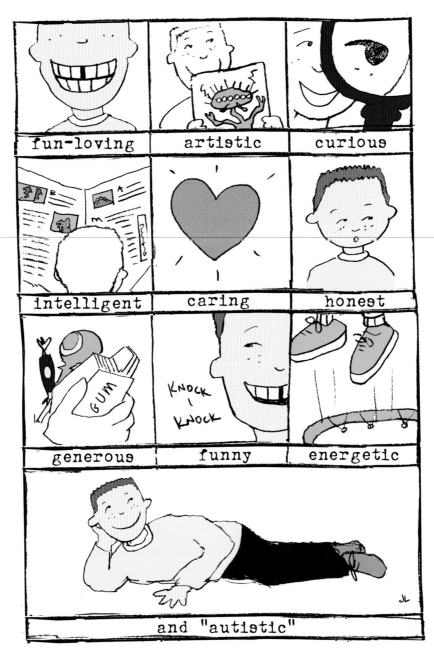

fun-loving | artistic | curious

intelligent | caring | honest

generous | funny | energetic

and "autistic"

"Autistic" just means
Matthew looks at the world
a little differently,

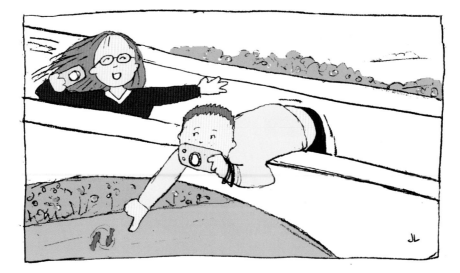

and, he isn't afraid
to be himself!

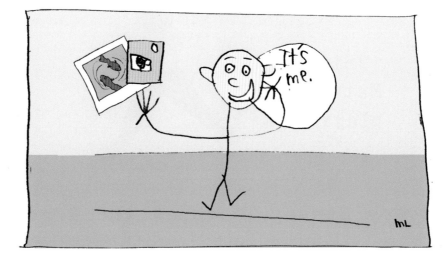

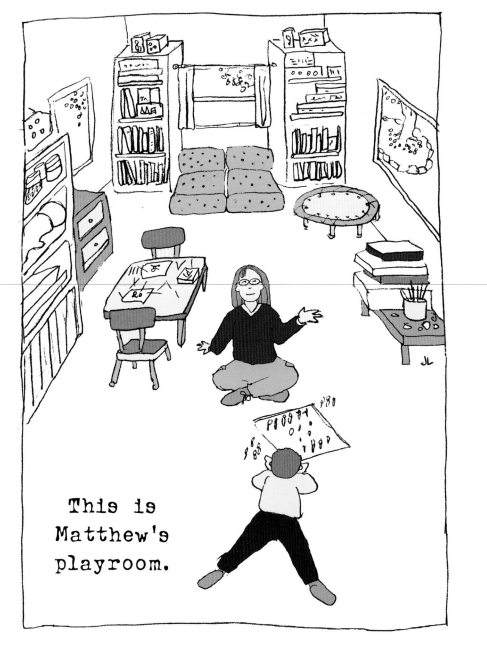

This is
Matthew's
playroom.

Every Sunday, Matthew and I get to
hang out together.

Matthew and I both like to draw,
so we each keep a sketchbook.

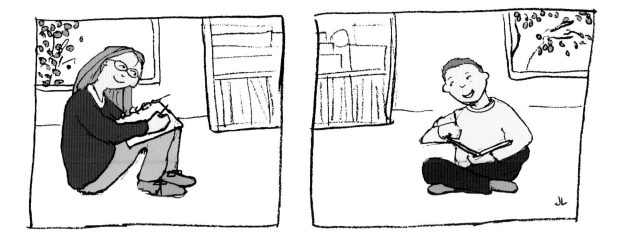

Sometimes, we swap books

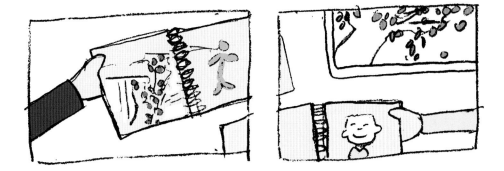

and tell each other
stories about our drawings.

This is one of Matthew's drawings.

Matthew says this is a troll,
who lives under a bridge.
This troll is not very nice.

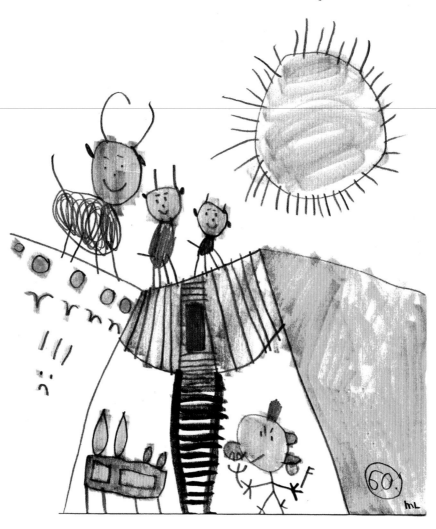

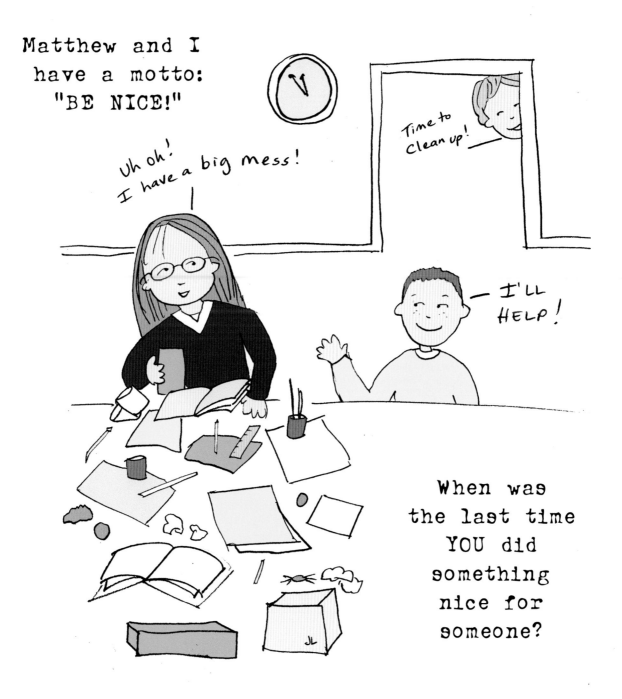

Sometimes people with autism
need a helping hand,

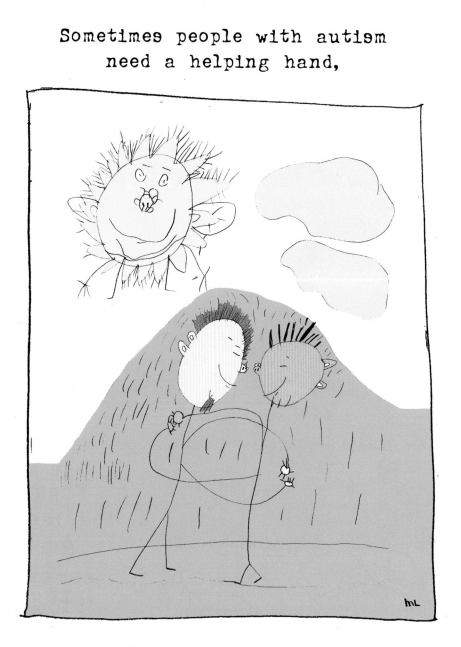

but if you pay attention,
they can teach you a lot.

People with autism have lots of
interesting thoughts, but they can't
always say them out loud.

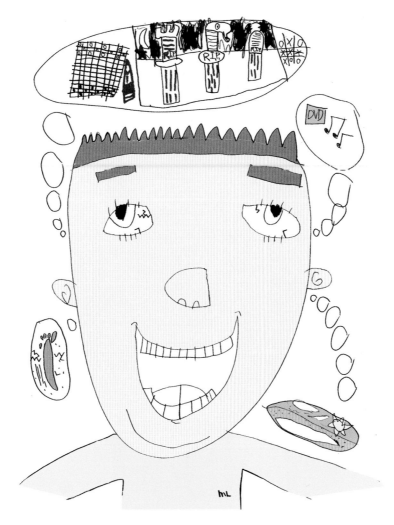

Matthew is very good at drawing
what's on his mind.

Matthew wonders, what if you were
a six-headed monster?

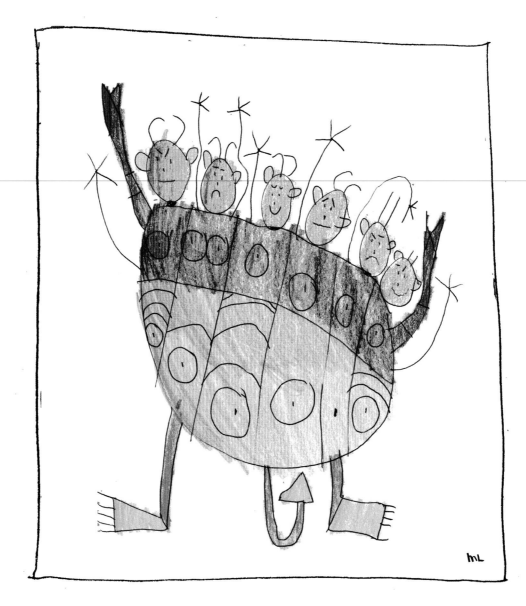

I wonder, what would it be like
to be in a room full of YOURSELF?

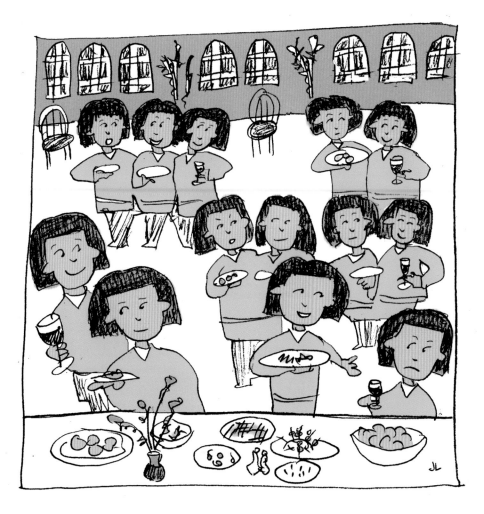

Are YOU a nice person
to be around?

Here are some of the things
Matthew and I love to think about.

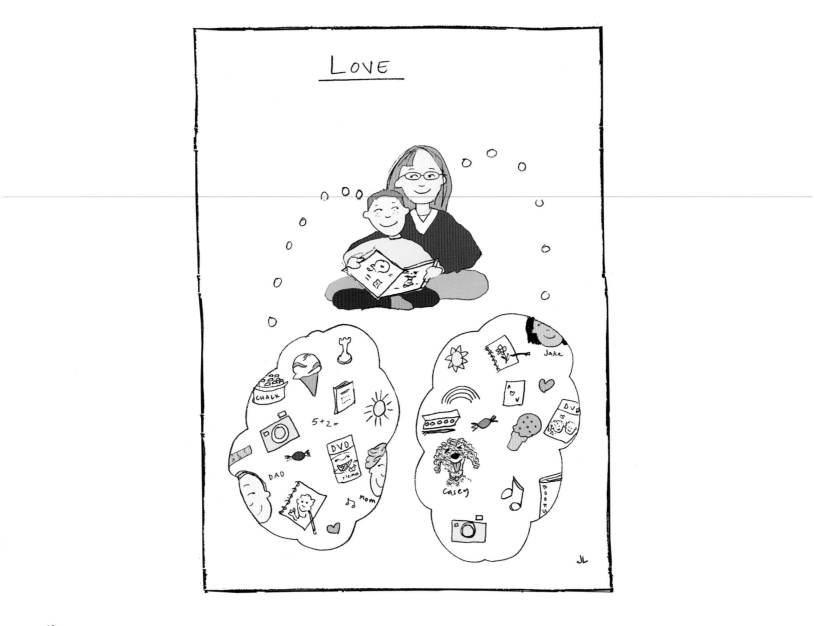

Matthew says he also loves math,
sea creatures, and waves.

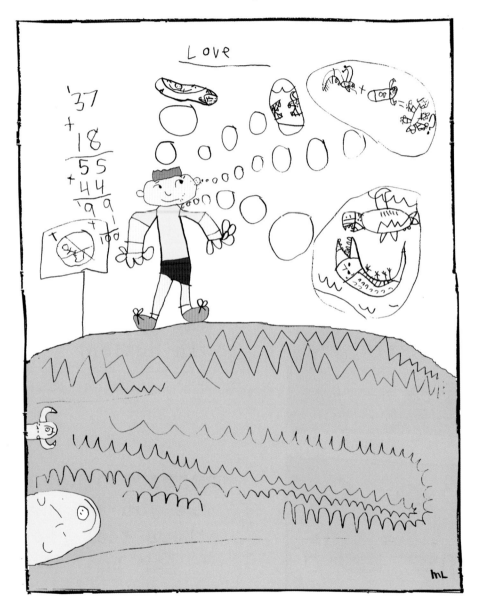

What do YOU love?

Sometimes Matthew and I talk about
what makes a good person.

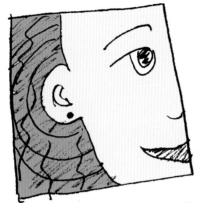

BE A GOOD LISTENER!
Pay attention and
save your comments
for your turn.

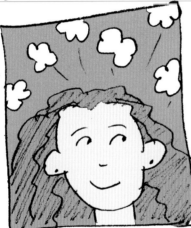

BE NICE!
In thoughts,
in words,
in action.

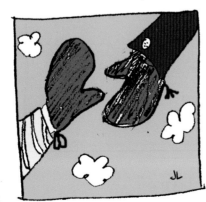

RESPECT OTHERS!
Are you making
others feel good
or bad?

Here are some more ideas.

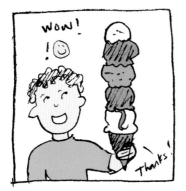

BE A GIVER!
Surprise people
by giving more
than they expect.

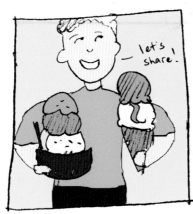

SHARE WHAT YOU HAVE!
Your good luck,
your love,
your feelings,
and your dreams.

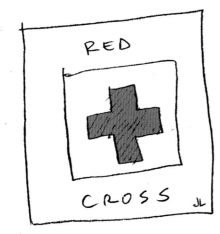

HELP OTHER PEOPLE!
Even a teeny,
tiny bit of
help is better
than none.

We think anyone can be whatever they want to be.

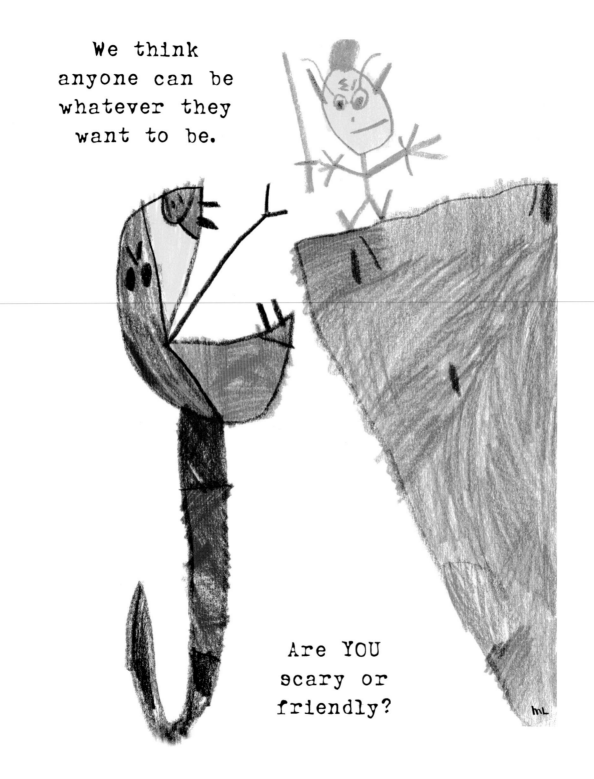

Are YOU scary or friendly?

Matthew and I talk about how everyone
has his own tone, or outlook on life.

Harsh Tone   &   Soft Tone

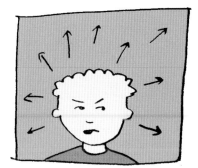 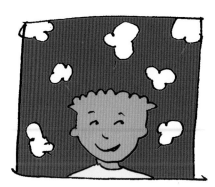

Ugg!   Yeah!

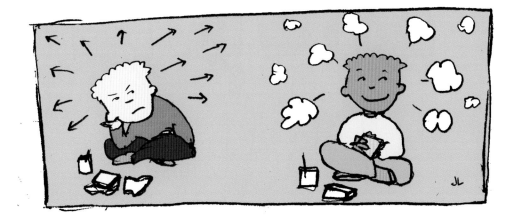

Who would you want to sit with?

I think everyone here on earth
has a mix of tones, and that is okay.

But heaven? Heaven's perfect!

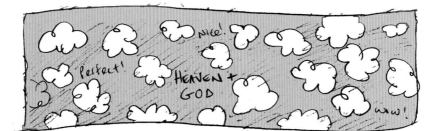

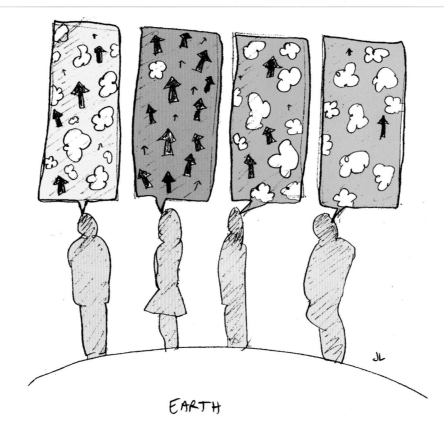

Silence can be a tone, too.

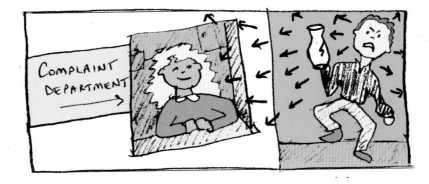

Silence can be good
(if you're listening).

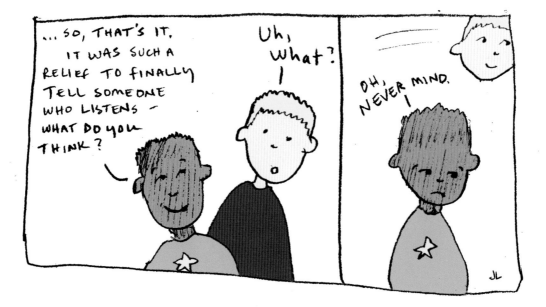

Silence can be bad
(if you're not listening).

Matthew draws a monster's tone
going from bad to worse.

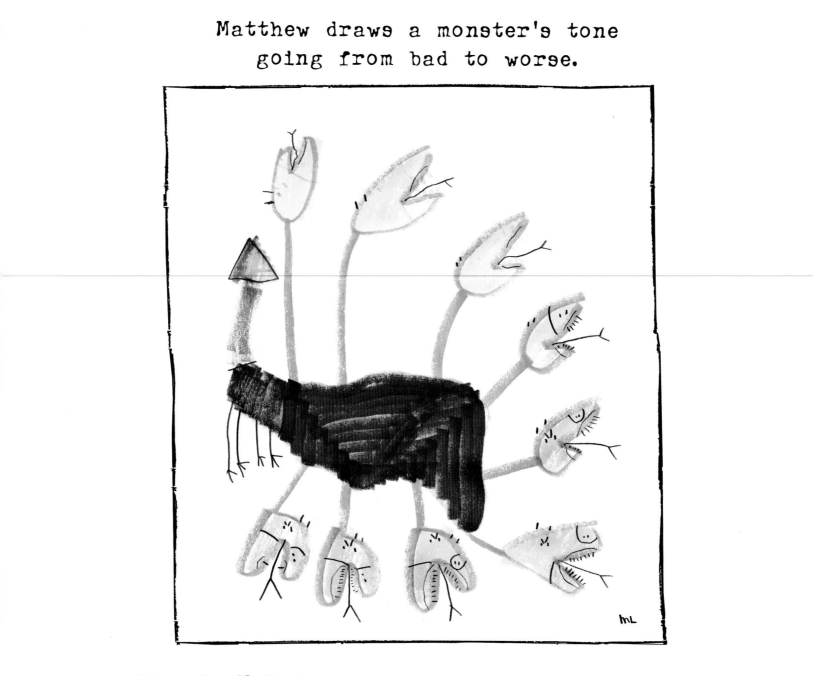

Why do YOU think the monster is so upset?

Maybe when someone you know
is acting like a monster,

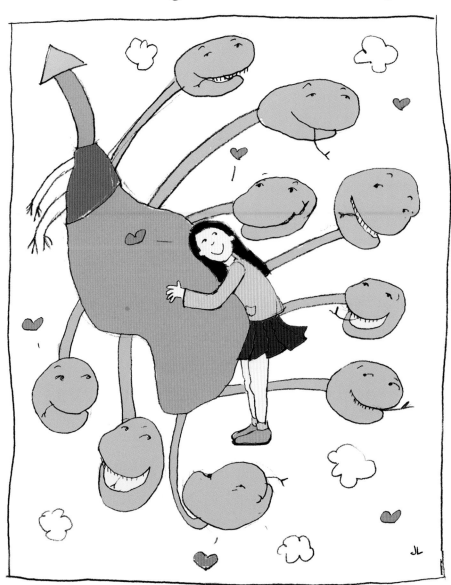

all she really needs is a hug!

One day Matthew and I were
talking about grandmothers.

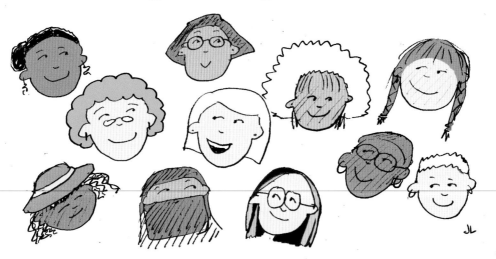

We wondered – if grandmothers
ruled the world,
would there be hugs
and cookies for everyone?

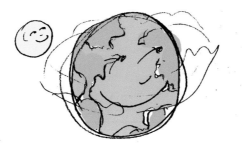

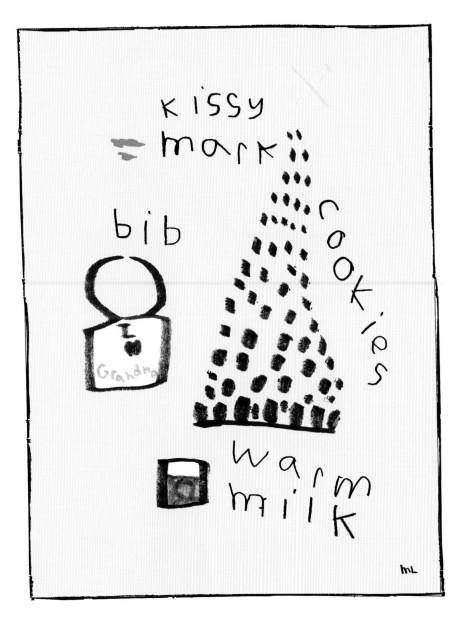

Matthew thinks that sounds
like a good idea!

Matthew and I think it's important
to respect other people's things
and their artwork.

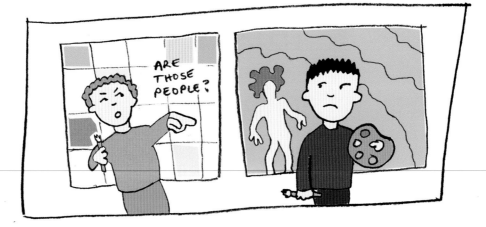

Don't say, "Mine is better!"

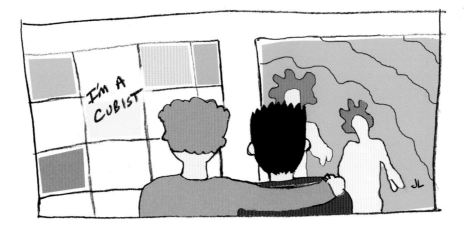

Instead, say "Look how different we are!"

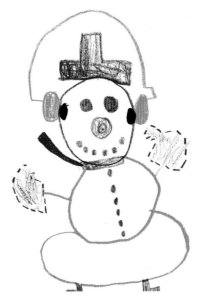

Everyone is always
having his or her own kind of day.

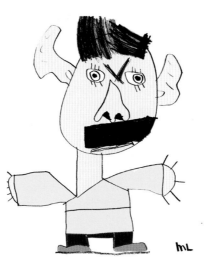

If you don't like the kind of day you're
having, you can change it!

How do you change your mind?

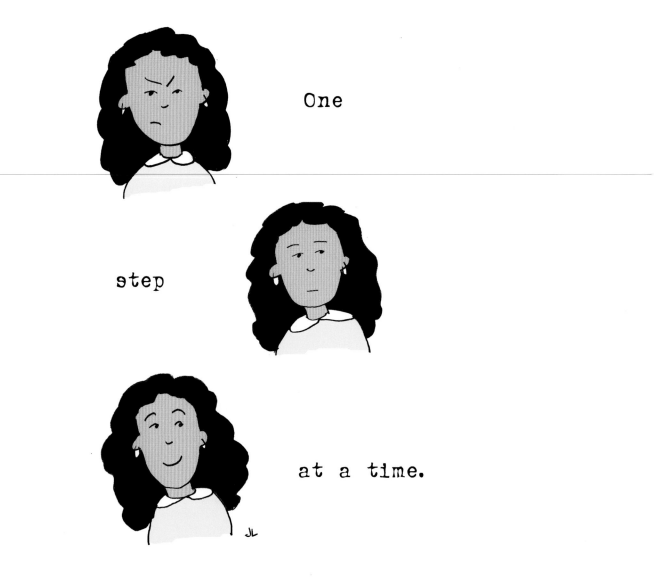

One

step

at a time.

If you look for a reason
to change your mind,

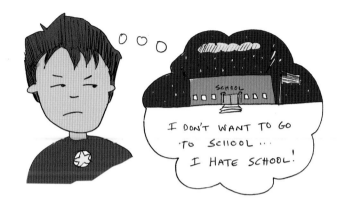

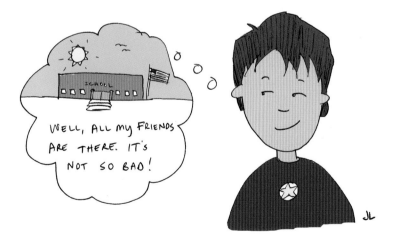

you can usually find one.

One day I asked Matthew,
how is life like a tree?

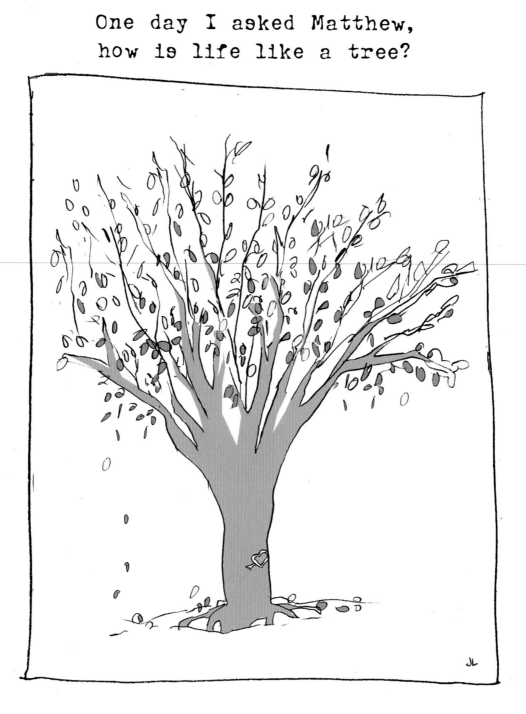

This picture is Matthew's answer.

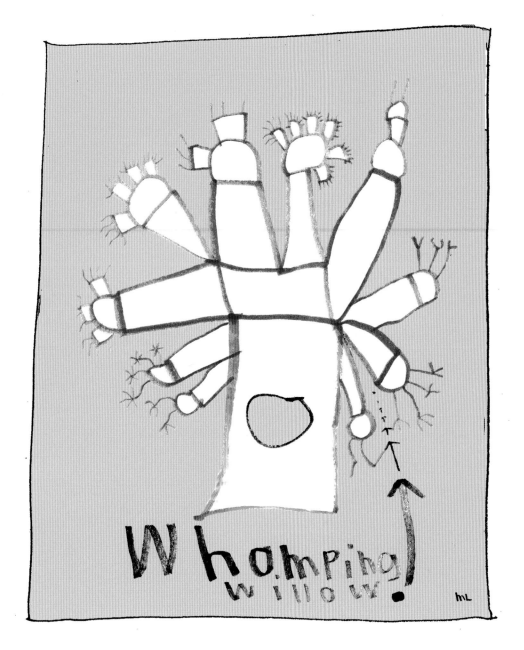

Sometimes Matthew asks me deep
questions like: "Where does God live?"

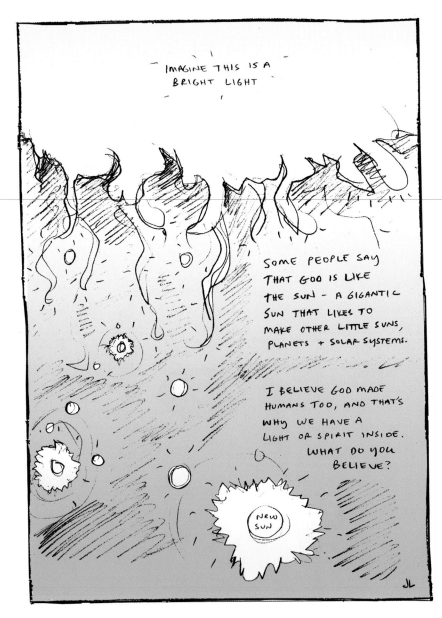

This is what Matthew imagines!

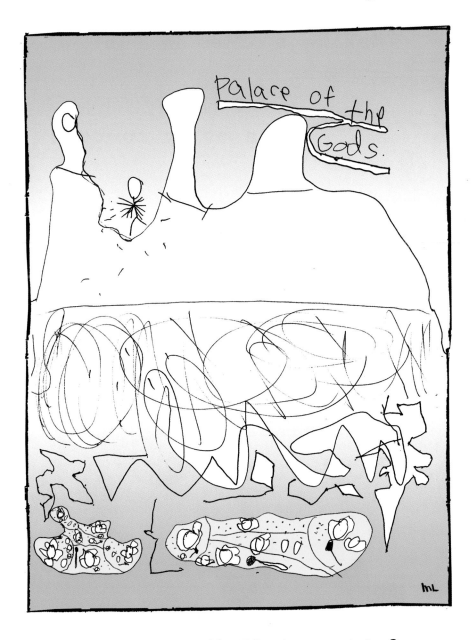

What are YOUR thoughts?

One day I asked Matthew what he wanted
to tell the world. He said:
"Making stories is fun!"

I bet YOU have
a story to tell!

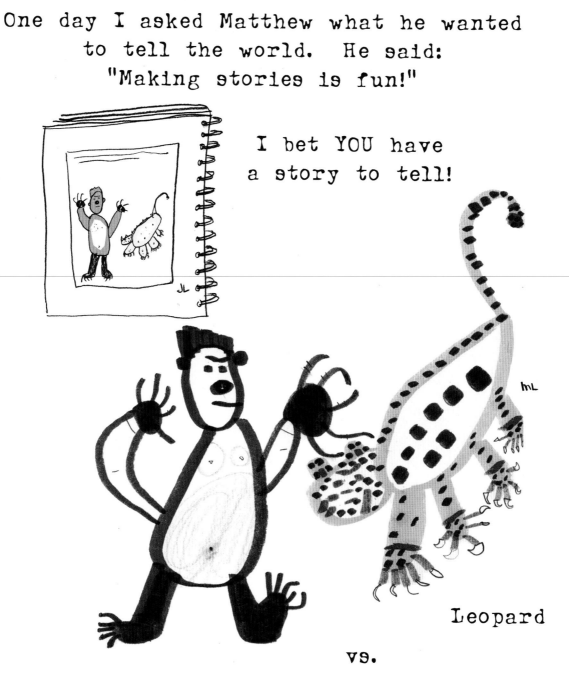

Gorilla

vs.

Leopard

Matthew says he wants to
be a professional photographer!

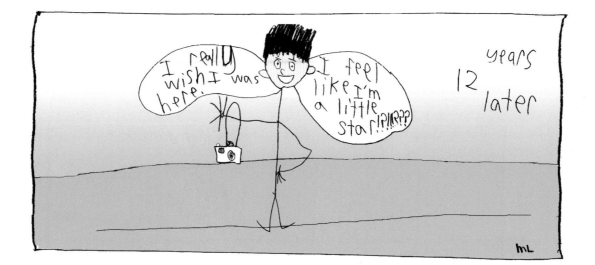

What would YOU like to be some day?

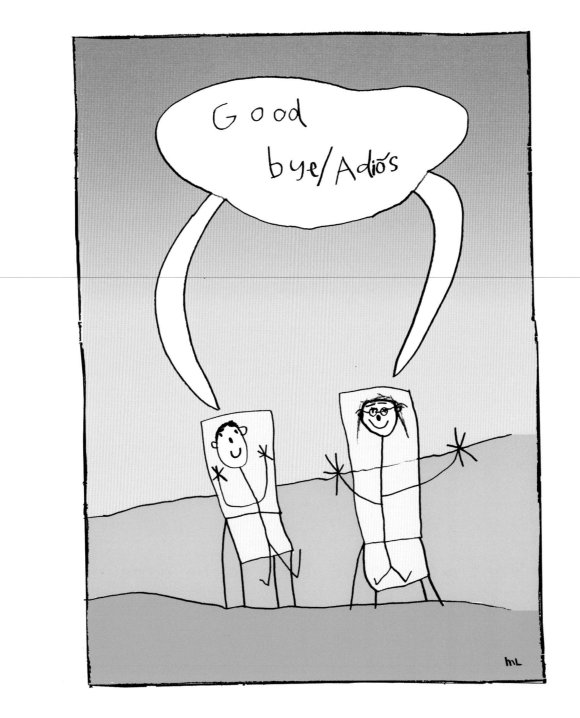

Thanks for hanging out with us!

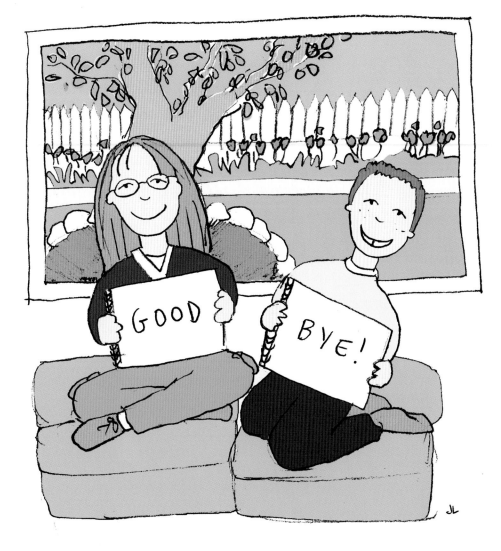

JEANETTE'S SKETCHBOOK TIPS

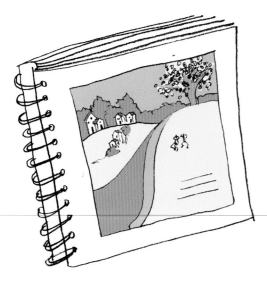

1. Find a nice sketchbook buddy to draw and share stories with.

2. Remember that all drawings are good, even if they're only stick people.

3. Draw a picture of yourself, or your buddy (and re-read #2).

4. Draw a story of something that really happened to you.

5. Draw a story out of your imagination.

6. Draw something that's important to you.

7. Draw a feeling or emotion.

8. Draw a picture of your biggest wish coming true.

9. Draw solutions to real-life problems or fears.

10. Always have fun and draw what you like!

I've found keeping dual sketchbooks is a wonderful way for Matthew and me to communicate. Since Matthew finds verbal communication difficult, drawing has given him an outlet to express what's on his mind in a fun, unrestricted, yet surprisingly concise way. Our drawings also spark conversation; we ask each other specific questions, and Matthew can often explain his drawings quite eloquently.

Topics Matthew and I tend to focus on include recognizing other people's emotions, and how to interact with others in an appropriate way. By assigning pictures and symbols to abstract concepts such as emotion, tone of voice, and silence, Matthew seems to understand them more completely. The drawings that served best as teaching tools were the ones drawn from real-life situations. The things Matthew learns through drawing seem to stick with him, and he never turns down the chance to draw something in the sketchbook!

Sundays with Matthew comes directly from our sketchbooks with some of our favorite topics.

J.L.

P.S. Always give your sketchbook buddy lots of encouragement, and remember – all drawings are expressions from the inside. Matthew will be the first to tell you, there is no such thing as a "wrong" drawing.

ABOUT THE AUTHORS

Matthew Lancelle is an eleven-year-old with autism. He likes to express himself through his artwork, and some of his favorite subjects are monsters and sea creatures. Matthew is also a photographer, who loves to read and look at picture books. He also likes chess, swimming, video games, watching movies and hanging out with his Mom Cindy, Dad Steve, sisters Elizabeth and Maggie, and brother David. Matthew says, "Making stories is fun!" Matthew attends Whitefish Bay Middle School in Whitefish Bay, Wisconsin.

Jeanette Lesada met Matthew in 2001 through the Wisconsin Early Autism Program. Despite funding cuts, Jeanette volunteers to visit Matthew every Sunday for art therapy. Jeanette says, "I try to encourage recycling positive thoughts. Many of our drawings come from real life, where we take a less-than-great situation and turn it into a positive one for next time." Jeanette has earned her B.F.A., has owned her own photography business, and is also a writer, Reiki master, and musician. She lives with her husband, Jake, an independent filmmaker and classic car painter, in Shorewood, Wisconsin.

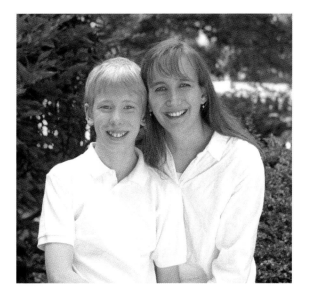

The Real Matthew & Jeanette!
photo by Sarah McEneany

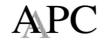

Autism Asperger Publishing Co.
P.O. Box 23173
Shawnee Mission, Kansas 66283-0173
www.asperger.net